I0446903

LOW SODIUM

SLOW COOKER

COOKBOOK

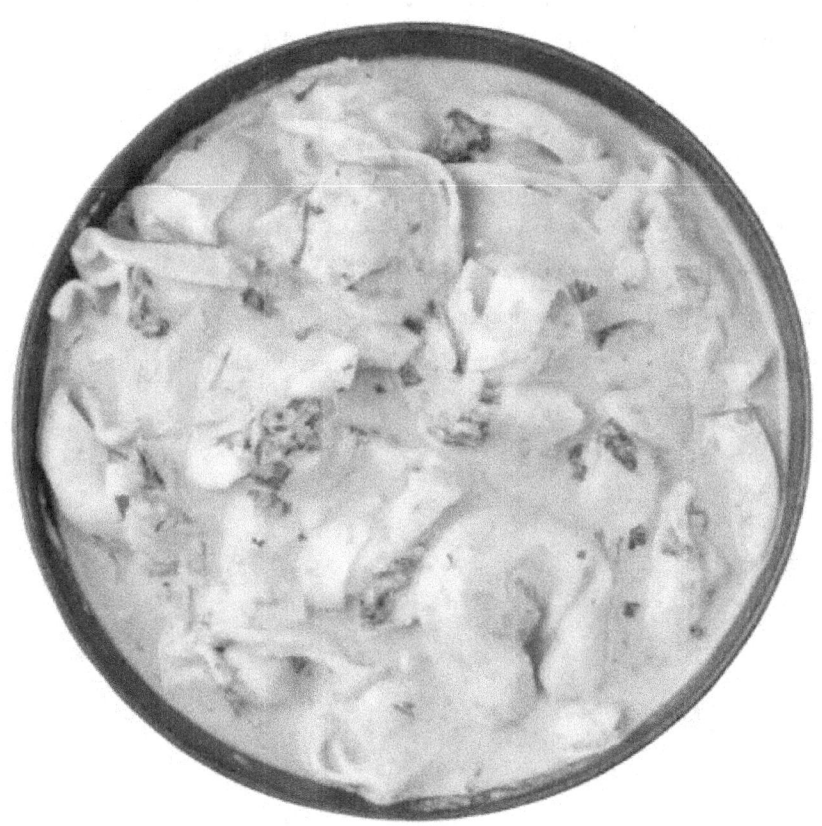

LORENE PEACHEY

Copyright © 2023 by Lorene Peachey

All rights reserved.

No part of this publication may be reproduced, stored in a retrieval system, or transmitted, in any form or by any means, electronic, mechanical, photocopying, recording or otherwise, without the prior written permission of the copyright holder.

This book is sold subject to the condition that it shall not, by way of trade or otherwise, be lent, re-sold, hired out or otherwise circulated without the publisher's prior consent in any form of binding or cover other than that in which it is published and without a similar condition including this condition being imposed on the subsequent purchaser.

The author has made every effort to ensure the accuracy and completeness of the Information contained in this book. However, the author and publisher assume no responsibility for errors, inaccuracies, omissions, or any inconsistency herein. Any slights of people, places or organizations are unintentional.

DISCLAIMER

The content within this book reflects my thoughts, experiences, and beliefs. It is meant for informational and entertainment purposes. While I have taken great care to provide accurate information, I cannot guarantee the absolute correctness or applicability of the content to every individual or situation. Please consult with relevant professionals for advice specific to your needs.

TABLE OF CONTENTS

INTRODUCTION

Hello, dear readers! I am Nutrionist Lorene Peachey, and I am thrilled to welcome you to a culinary journey that changed my life and the lives of countless others. Today, I want to share with you a deeply personal experience that led me to create a cookbook that has become a beacon of hope for those seeking a delicious, heart-healthy lifestyle.

It all began with a phone call from my dear friend, Sarah Johnson. We shared countless memories, from college shenanigans to navigating the rollercoaster of adulthood. Sarah, however, faced a silent battle—high blood pressure. Despite trying various cookbooks and diets, her quest for flavourful yet heart-healthy meals had proven futile.

As a nutritionist, I couldn't stand idly by while my friend struggled. That's when I decided to put my skills to the test. I delved into the world of low-sodium slow cooking, determined to create recipes that not only met her dietary needs but also tantalized her taste buds. Little did I know that this experiment would lead to the creation of the cookbook you now hold in your hands.

It's a chilly Sunday afternoon, the aroma of slow-cooked goodness wafting through the air. The doorbell rings, and there stands Sarah, her eyes widened by the savory symphony in my kitchen. One bite, and she was hooked. The recipes in this cookbook transformed her culinary experience, proving that low sodium didn't mean sacrificing flavour.

But let's dive deeper into the why—why does a low-sodium diet matter, and what are the consequences of neglecting it?

Consider for a moment the effects of a high-sodium diet on our bodies. The silent saboteur, sodium, often lurks in processed foods, ready to wreak havoc on our health. High blood pressure, bloating, and an increased risk of heart disease are just the tip of the iceberg. I'm sure many of you, like me, have questioned whether there's a way to enjoy food without jeopardizing our well-being.

That's where this cookbook steps in, offering you not just a collection of recipes but a lifeline to a healthier, more vibrant you. As you embark on this culinary adventure, ask yourself: How would it feel to Savor delicious meals without compromising on health? Can you imagine the joy of nourishing your body and soul simultaneously?

Let me assure you, the benefits of a low-sodium diet extend far beyond the kitchen. Weight management, reduced risk of chronic diseases, and increased energy levels are just a few of the perks awaiting you. It's not just about eating; it's about embracing a lifestyle that Honors your well-being.

As I pen down these words, I am reminded of the countless success stories from individuals who've embraced the recipes within these pages. From John, who saw his blood pressure normalize, to Emily, a young mother who rediscovered the joy of cooking for her family without compromising on health—each story is a testament to the transformative power of conscious eating.

Now, you might be wondering, "What sets this cookbook apart from the rest?" The answer lies not just in the recipes but in the journey, we embark upon together. This isn't a mere collection of instructions; it's a guide to a healthier, more flavourful life. With each turn of the page, you'll discover the joy of creating mouthwatering dishes that love your heart back.

Imagine a dinner table adorned with slow-cooked wonders—tender pot roasts, aromatic stews, and delectable desserts—all crafted with your well-being in mind. The beauty of this cookbook lies not just in its ability to transform ingredients but in its power to transform lives.

As you flip through these pages, allow yourself to be captivated by the possibilities. Picture the smiles around your table as loved one's Savor meals that nurture their bodies. Envision a future where your kitchen becomes a sanctuary of health, and every bite is a step towards a more vibrant you.

So, my dear friends, are you ready to embark on this journey with me? Can you feel the excitement bubbling within, urging you to explore the world of low-sodium slow cooking? I invite you to Savor the stories, Flavors, and moments that await you in the pages of this cookbook. Let it be a companion on your path to wellness, reminding you that health and happiness are within reach—one delicious meal at a time.

Welcome to a world where your journey to a healthier you is as flavourful as it is fulfilling. Let the adventure begin!

Contact the Author

Thank you for reading my book! I would love to hear from you, whether you have feedback, questions, or just want to share your thoughts. Your feedback means a lot to me and helps me improve as a writer.

Please don't hesitate to reach out to me through

lorenepeachey@gmail.com

I look forward to connecting with my readers and appreciate your support in this literary journey. Your thoughts and comments are valuable to me.

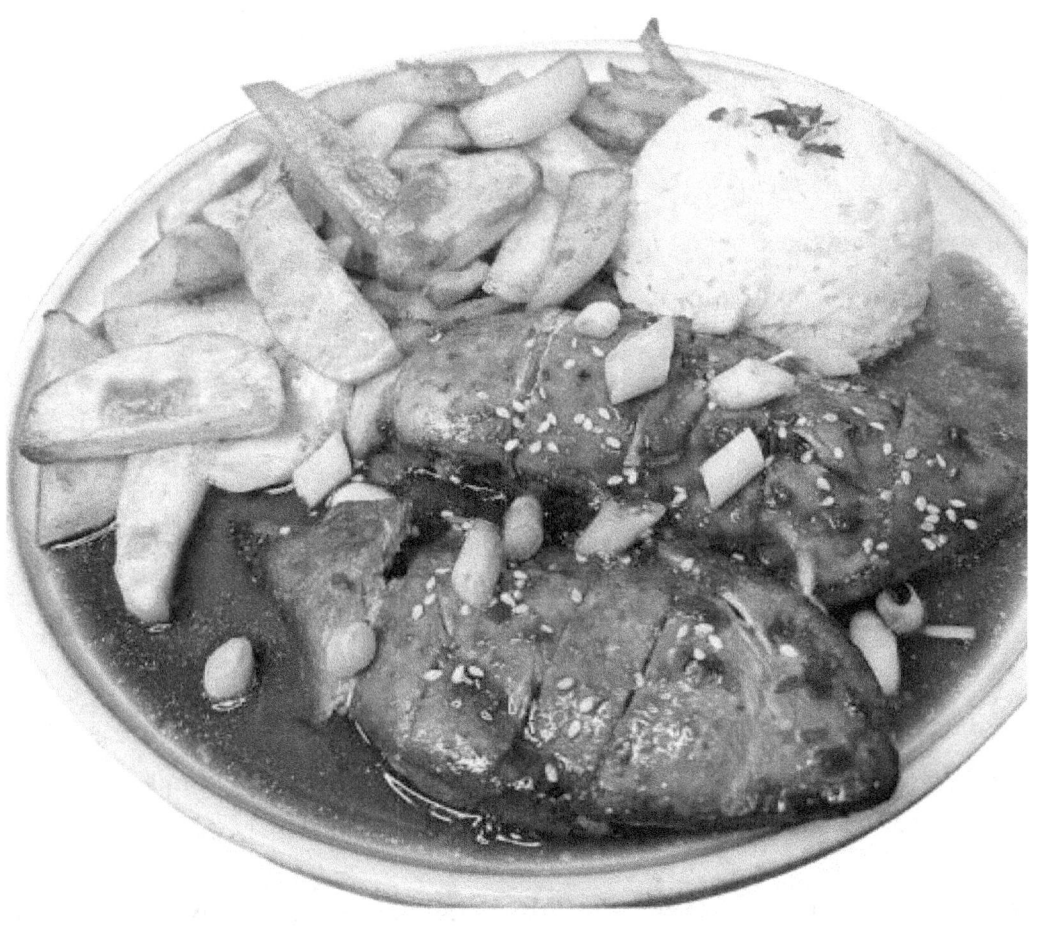

CHAPTER 1

LOW SODIUM COOKING

In the realm of healthy eating, a low sodium diet has gained prominence for its numerous benefits. Reducing sodium intake can contribute to better heart health, lower blood pressure, and overall well-being. One effective way to embark on this journey is by adopting low sodium cooking practices. In this Cookbook, we'll explore the advantages of a low sodium diet and provide valuable tips for minimizing salt content in slow cooker recipes.

Benefits of a Low Sodium Diet:

Heart Health: High sodium intake is often linked to hypertension, which is a major risk factor for heart disease. By embracing a low sodium diet, individuals can support cardiovascular health and reduce the likelihood of developing heart-related conditions.

Blood Pressure Management: Sodium plays a significant role in regulating blood pressure. A low sodium diet helps maintain optimal blood pressure levels, reducing the strain on the heart and arteries.

Kidney Function: Excessive sodium can contribute to kidney damage over time. A low sodium diet supports kidney function by preventing the accumulation of harmful substances and reducing the risk of kidney-related issues.

Fluid Balance: Sodium influences fluid balance in the body. Reducing sodium intake helps prevent water retention, decreasing the risk of swelling and edema.

Improved Overall Well-being: A low sodium diet is associated with better overall health. It can lead to increased energy levels, improved digestion, and a reduced risk of chronic diseases.

Tips for Reducing Sodium in Slow Cooker Recipes:

Choose Fresh Ingredients: Opt for fresh, whole ingredients to control the sodium content from the start. Fresh vegetables, lean meats, and herbs can add natural flavor without relying on salt.

Limit Processed Ingredients: Processed foods often contain high levels of sodium. Minimize the use of canned soups, broths, and pre-packaged sauces in slow cooker recipes. Instead, prepare your own flavorful alternatives.

Herbs and Spices: Experiment with herbs and spices to enhance the taste of your dishes. Utilize garlic, onion, basil, oregano, and other herbs to create a savory profile without the need for excessive salt.

Use Citrus Juices and Vinegar: Citrus juices and vinegar can add a tangy flavor to your recipes, reducing the reliance on salt. Consider marinating meats in citrus-based solutions for added tenderness and taste.

Gradual Reduction: If you're accustomed to a higher sodium diet, gradually reduce the salt in your recipes. This allows your taste buds to adjust, making the transition to lower sodium levels more manageable.

CHAPTER 1

SLOW COOKER BASICS

Slow cookers, also known as crockpots, have become indispensable kitchen companions for those seeking convenient and flavorful meals. This guide explores the fundamental aspects of slow cooking, from selecting the right appliance to essential tools and ingredients that make the process seamless.

Choosing the Right Slow Cooker:

Size Matters: Slow cookers come in various sizes, typically measured in quarts. Consider the number of people you'll be serving and the type of meals you plan to prepare. Smaller units are ideal for individuals or couples, while larger families may benefit from 6 to 8-quart models.

Settings and Features: Opt for a slow cooker with adjustable temperature settings, including low and high heat options. Some models even offer programmable timers, allowing for precise control over cooking times. Keep an eye out for removable, dishwasher-safe inserts for easy cleanup.

Shape Considerations: Slow cookers come in oval and round shapes. Oval models are ideal for cooking large cuts of meat and accommodating awkwardly shaped ingredients, while round ones work well for soups, stews, and casseroles.

Budget and Brand: Determine your budget and explore reputable brands. While there are budget-friendly options, investing in a quality slow cooker can ensure durability and consistent performance over time.

Essential Tools and Ingredients:

Quality Meats: Choose cuts of meat suitable for slow cooking, such as beef chuck, pork shoulder, or chicken thighs. These cuts become tender and flavorful during the slow cooking process.

Fresh Vegetables: Incorporate a variety of fresh vegetables for added nutrition and taste. Root vegetables like carrots and potatoes hold up well to extended cooking times.

Broths and Liquids: Use flavorful broths, stocks, or sauces to enhance the taste of your dishes. Opt for low-sodium versions to maintain control over the overall sodium content.

Herbs and Spices: Elevate your slow cooker recipes with a blend of herbs and spices. Common choices include thyme, rosemary, garlic, and bay leaves. Experiment to find combinations that suit your palate.

Thickening Agents: If you desire a thicker consistency for your dishes, consider using ingredients like flour, cornstarch, or tomato paste. Add them towards the end of the cooking time to achieve the desired texture.

Searing for Flavor: While not essential, searing meats before placing them in the slow cooker can enhance the flavor and appearance of the final dish. It adds a depth of richness by caramelizing the surface of the meat.

CHAPTER 3

BREAKFAST DELIGHTS

Quinoa Breakfast Bowl

Cooking Time: 4 hours on low

Servings: 4

Ingredients:

- ❖ 1 cup quinoa, rinsed.
- ❖ 2 cups almond milk (low sodium)
- ❖ 1 cup fresh berries
- ❖ 1/4 cup chopped nuts.
- ❖ 1 teaspoon vanilla extract

Instructions:

1. Combine quinoa, almond milk, and vanilla extract in the slow cooker.
2. Cook on low for 4 hours.
3. Serve topped with fresh berries and chopped nuts.

Nutritional Information:

300 calories, 45g carbs, 10g protein, 8g fat, 7g fiber

Start your day with a protein-packed quinoa bowl, loaded with antioxidants from fresh berries.

Vegetable Frittata

Cooking Time: 3 hours on low

Servings: 6

Ingredients:

- ❖ 8 eggs, beaten.
- ❖ 1 cup low-fat cheese, shredded.
- ❖ 1 cup spinach, chopped.
- ❖ 1 bell pepper, diced.
- ❖ 1/2 cup cherry tomatoes, halved.

Instructions:

1. Grease the slow cooker with cooking spray.
2. Mix eggs, cheese, spinach, bell pepper, and tomatoes in a bowl.
3. Pour the mixture into the slow cooker and cook on low for 3 hours.

Nutritional Information:

200 calories, 10g carbs, 15g protein, 12g fat, 3g fiber

Indulge in a savory frittata, packed with veggies and protein to keep you energized throughout the morning.

Oatmeal with Apples and Cinnamon

Cooking Time: 6 hours on low

Servings: 4

Ingredients:

- ❖ 2 cups steel-cut oats
- ❖ 4 cups water
- ❖ 2 apples, diced.
- ❖ 1 teaspoon cinnamon
- ❖ 1/4 cup maple syrup (optional)

Instructions:

1. Combine oats, water, apples, and cinnamon in the slow cooker.
2. Cook on low for 6 hours.
3. Sweeten with maple syrup if desired before serving.

Nutritional Information:

250 calories, 50g carbs, 7g protein, 3g fat, 8g fiber

Wake up to the aroma of cinnamon-infused oatmeal with the natural sweetness of apples.

Sweet Potato and Turkey Sausage Casserole

Cooking Time: 5 hours on low

Servings: 5

Ingredients:

- ❖ 2 sweet potatoes peeled and diced.
- ❖ 1 pound low-sodium turkey sausage, crumbled.
- ❖ 1 onion, chopped.
- ❖ 1 bell pepper, diced.
- ❖ 8 eggs, beaten.

Instructions:

1. Layer sweet potatoes, turkey sausage, onion, and bell pepper in the slow cooker.
2. Pour beaten eggs over the layers.
3. Cook on low for 5 hours.

Nutritional Information:

280 calories, 25g carbs, 20g protein, 12g fat, 5g fiber

Enjoy a hearty casserole that combines the goodness of sweet potatoes and lean turkey sausage.

Chia Seed Pudding

Cooking Time: 2 hours on low

Servings: 4

Ingredients:

- ❖ 1/2 cup chia seeds
- ❖ 2 cups unsweetened almond milk (low sodium)
- ❖ 1 teaspoon vanilla extract
- ❖ 1 tablespoon honey
- ❖ Fresh fruit for topping

Instructions:

1. Mix chia seeds, almond milk, vanilla extract, and honey in the slow cooker.
2. Cook on low for 2 hours, stirring occasionally.
3. Serve topped with fresh fruit.

Nutritional Information:

180 calories, 20g carbs, 5g protein, 10g fat, 8g fiber

Indulge in a nutritious chia seed pudding, a delightful and low-sodium alternative to traditional breakfast options.

Blueberry Almond Oat Bars

Cooking Time: 4 hours on low

Servings: 8

Ingredients:

- ❖ 2 cups rolled oats.
- ❖ 1 cup almond butter
- ❖ 1/2 cup honey
- ❖ 1/2 cup unsweetened applesauce
- ❖ 1 cup fresh blueberries

Instructions:

1. Mix oats, almond butter, honey, and applesauce in a bowl.
2. Fold in fresh blueberries.
3. Press the mixture into the slow cooker and cook on low for 4 hours.

Nutritional Information:

220 calories, 30g carbs, 6g protein, 10g fat, 4g fiber

Satisfy your sweet tooth with these blueberry almond oat bars, a guilt-free breakfast treat.

Spinach and Mushroom Egg Casserole

Cooking Time: 3 hours on low

Servings: 6

Ingredients:

- ❖ 8 eggs, beaten.
- ❖ 1 cup low-fat feta cheese, crumbled.
- ❖ 2 cups spinach, chopped.
- ❖ 1 cup mushrooms, sliced.
- ❖ 1 teaspoon garlic powder

Instructions:

1. Grease the slow cooker with cooking spray.
2. Mix eggs, feta, spinach, mushrooms, and garlic powder in a bowl.
3. Pour the mixture into the slow cooker and cook on low for 3 hours.

Nutritional Information:

180 calories, 8g carbs, 15g protein, 10g fat, 2g fiber

Fuel your morning with a protein-packed egg casserole featuring the earthy flavors of spinach and mushrooms.

Cranberry Orange Steel-Cut Oats

Cooking Time: 6 hours on low

Servings: 4

Ingredients:

- ❖ 1 cup steel-cut oats
- ❖ 4 cups water
- ❖ 1/2 cup dried cranberries
- ❖ Zest of one orange
- ❖ 1/4 cup maple syrup (optional)

Instructions:

1. Combine oats, water, cranberries, and orange zest in the slow cooker.
2. Cook on low for 6 hours.
3. Sweeten with maple syrup if desired before serving.

Nutritional Information:

240 calories, 45g carbs, 7g protein, 4g fat, 6g fiber

Start your day with the delightful combination of cranberries and orange zest in these nutritious steel-cut oats.

Turkey and Vegetable Breakfast Burrito Filling

Cooking Time: 4 hours on low

Servings: 6

Ingredients:

- ❖ 1 pound ground turkey (93% lean)
- ❖ 1 onion, chopped.
- ❖ 1 bell pepper, diced.
- ❖ 1 zucchini, shredded.
- ❖ 1 teaspoon cumin

Instructions:

1. Cook ground turkey in a skillet until browned, transfer to the slow cooker.
2. Add chopped onion, diced bell pepper, shredded zucchini, and cumin to the slow cooker.
3. Cook on low for 4 hours.

Nutritional Information:

220 calories, 15g carbs, 20g protein, 10g fat, 3g fiber

Create a savory breakfast burrito filling with lean turkey and an array of colorful veggies.

Banana Walnut Breakfast Quinoa

Cooking Time: 3 hours on low

Servings: 4

Ingredients:

- ❖ 1 cup quinoa, rinsed.
- ❖ 2 cups coconut milk (low sodium)
- ❖ 2 ripe bananas, mashed.
- ❖ 1/2 cup chopped walnuts.
- ❖ 1 tablespoon honey

Instructions:

1. Combine quinoa, coconut milk, mashed bananas, and chopped walnuts in the slow cooker.
2. Cook on low for 3 hours.
3. Drizzle with honey before serving.

Nutritional Information:

280 calories, 40g carbs, 8g protein, 10g fat, 6g fiber

Indulge in the rich flavors of banana and walnut in this satisfying and low-sodium breakfast quinoa.

CHAPTER 4

APPETIZERS AND SNACKS

Spicy Black Bean Dip

Cooking Time: 3 hours on low

Servings: 8

Ingredients:

- ❖ 2 cans (15 oz each) low-sodium black beans, drained and rinsed
- ❖ 1 cup salsa
- ❖ 1 teaspoon cumin
- ❖ 1/2 teaspoon chili powder
- ❖ 1 cup low-fat shredded cheese

Instructions:

1. Combine black beans, salsa, cumin, and chili powder in the slow cooker.
2. Cook on low for 3 hours.
3. Top with shredded cheese before serving.

Nutritional Information:

120 calories, 15g carbs, 8g protein, 4g fat, 6g fiber

Kick off your gathering with this flavorful and protein-packed black bean dip, perfect for dipping your favorite veggies.

Mango Salsa Chicken Wings

Cooking Time: 4 hours on low

Servings: 12

Ingredients:

- ❖ 2 lbs. chicken wings
- ❖ 1 cup mango, diced.
- ❖ 1/2 cup red onion finely chopped.
- ❖ 1/4 cup cilantro, chopped.
- ❖ 1 teaspoon cayenne pepper

Instructions:

1. Place chicken wings in the slow cooker.
2. In a bowl, mix mango, red onion, cilantro, and cayenne pepper; pour over the chicken.
3. Cook on low for 4 hours.

Nutritional Information:

180 calories, 5g carbs, 15g protein, 10g fat, 1g fiber

Elevate your game day snacks with these succulent mango salsa chicken wings, a sweet and spicy twist on a classic.

Cauliflower and Artichoke Dip

Cooking Time: 2 hours on low

Servings: 10

Ingredients:

- ❖ 1 head cauliflower, chopped.
- ❖ 1 can (14 oz) artichoke hearts drained and chopped.
- ❖ 1 cup Greek yogurt
- ❖ 1 cup low-fat mayonnaise
- ❖ 1 cup grated Parmesan cheese.

Instructions:

1. Combine cauliflower, artichoke hearts, Greek yogurt, mayonnaise, and Parmesan cheese in the slow cooker.
2. Cook on low for 2 hours.
3. Stir well before serving.

Nutritional Information:

150 calories, 8g carbs, 10g protein, 8g fat, 3g fiber

Dive into a guilt-free indulgence with this creamy cauliflower and artichoke dip, a crowd-pleasing low-sodium option.

Teriyaki Turkey Meatballs

Cooking Time: 3 hours on low

Servings: 20

Ingredients:

- ❖ 1 lb ground turkey (93% lean)
- ❖ 1/2 cup breadcrumbs
- ❖ 1/4 cup low-sodium soy sauce
- ❖ 1/4 cup hoisin sauce
- ❖ 2 teaspoons ginger, minced.

Instructions:

1. In a bowl, mix ground turkey, breadcrumbs, soy sauce, hoisin sauce, and ginger.
2. Shape into meatballs and place in the slow cooker.
3. Cook on low for 3 hours.

Nutritional Information:

90 calories, 5g carbs, 8g protein, 4g fat, 1g fiber

Savor the flavor of teriyaki with these lean turkey meatballs, a savory and protein-packed party snack.

Vegetarian Lentil Soup

Cooking Time: 4 hours on low

Servings: 8

Ingredients:

- ❖ 1 cup dried lentils, rinsed.
- ❖ 2 carrots, diced.
- ❖ 2 celery stalks, diced.
- ❖ 1 onion, chopped.
- ❖ 3 cloves garlic, minced.

Instructions:

1. Combine lentils, carrots, celery, onion, and garlic in the slow cooker.
2. Add water to cover the ingredients and cook on low for 4 hours.
3. Season with salt and pepper to taste before serving.

Nutritional Information:

120 calories, 20g carbs, 8g protein, 1g fat, 8g fiber

Warm up your guests with a wholesome and low-sodium lentil soup, perfect for any gathering.

Zesty Shrimp and Avocado Ceviche

Cooking Time: 1 hour on low

Servings: 6

Ingredients:

- ❖ 1 lb cooked shrimp, peeled and deveined.
- ❖ 2 avocados, diced.
- ❖ 1 cup cherry tomatoes, halved.
- ❖ 1/2 red onion finely chopped.
- ❖ 1/4 cup fresh cilantro, chopped.

Instructions:

1. Mix shrimp, avocados, cherry tomatoes, red onion, and cilantro in the slow cooker.
2. Refrigerate for at least 1 hour before serving.

Nutritional Information:

160 calories, 10g carbs, 15g protein, 8g fat, 5g fiber

Satisfy your cravings with this refreshing shrimp and avocado ceviche, a low-sodium twist on a classic appetizer.

Sesame Ginger Edamame

Cooking Time: 2 hours on low

Servings: 4

Ingredients:

- ❖ 2 cups frozen edamame
- ❖ 2 tablespoons low-sodium soy sauce
- ❖ 1 tablespoon sesame oil
- ❖ 1 teaspoon grated ginger
- ❖ 1 teaspoon sesame seeds

Instructions:

1. Place edamame in the slow cooker.
2. In a bowl, mix soy sauce, sesame oil, ginger, and sesame seeds; pour over the edamame.
3. Cook on low for 2 hours.

Nutritional Information:

120 calories, 8g carbs, 10g protein, 6g fat, 4g fiber

Elevate your snack game with these sesame ginger edamame, a flavorful and protein-rich option for mindful munching.

Cucumber and Hummus Stuffed Cherry Tomatoes

Cooking Time: 1 hour on low

Servings: 12

Ingredients:

- ❖ 24 cherry tomatoes
- ❖ 1 cucumber finely diced.
- ❖ 1 cup hummus (low sodium)
- ❖ Fresh parsley for garnish

Instructions:

1. Cut a small portion off the bottom of each cherry tomato to create a stable base.
2. Scoop out the seeds and fill each tomato with hummus.
3. Top with diced cucumber and garnish with fresh parsley.

Nutritional Information:

50 calories, 6g carbs, 2g protein, 3g fat, 2g fiber

Enjoy a burst of freshness with these bite-sized cucumber and hummus stuffed cherry tomatoes, perfect for guilt-free snacking.

Italian Herb Roasted Nuts

Cooking Time: 2 hours on low

Servings: 10

Ingredients:

- ❖ 2 cups mixed nuts (almonds, walnuts, cashews)
- ❖ 2 tablespoons olive oil
- ❖ 1 tablespoon Italian herb seasoning
- ❖ 1 teaspoon garlic powder

Instructions:

1. Toss mixed nuts with olive oil, Italian herb seasoning, and garlic powder.
2. Spread on the slow cooker and cook on low for 2 hours, stirring occasionally.

Nutritional Information:

180 calories, 8g carbs, 6g protein, 15g fat, 3g fiber

Elevate your nut game with these Italian herb-roasted nuts, a savory and heart-healthy snack option.

Stuffed Bell Peppers with Quinoa and Black Beans

Cooking Time: 3 hours on low

Servings: 8

Ingredients:

- ❖ 4 bell peppers halved and seeds removed.
- ❖ 1 cup cooked quinoa
- ❖ 1 can (15 oz) low-sodium black beans, drained and rinsed
- ❖ 1 cup corn kernels
- ❖ 1 teaspoon cumin

Instructions:

1. Mix cooked quinoa, black beans, corn, and cumin in a bowl.
2. Stuff each bell pepper in half with the quinoa mixture.
3. Place in the slow cooker and cook on low for 3 hours.

Nutritional Information:

160 calories, 30g carbs, 8g protein, 2g fat, 6g fiber

Transform bell peppers into a delicious and nutritious snack with these stuffed peppers, filled with quinoa and black beans.

CHAPTER 4

SOUPS AND STEWS

Vegetarian Minestrone Soup

Cooking Time: 4 hours on low

Servings: 6

Ingredients:

- ❖ 4 cups vegetable broth (low sodium)
- ❖ 1 can (15 oz) diced tomatoes, undrained.
- ❖ 2 carrots, diced.
- ❖ 2 celery stalks, chopped.
- ❖ 1 zucchini, sliced.
- ❖ 1 cup green beans, chopped.
- ❖ 1 cup kidney beans drained and rinsed.
- ❖ 1 cup whole wheat pasta
- ❖ 1 teaspoon Italian seasoning

Instructions:

1. Combine all ingredients in the slow cooker.

2. Cook on low for 4 hours.

3. Season with salt and pepper to taste before serving.

Nutritional Information:

180 calories, 35g carbs, 8g protein, 1g fat, 7g fiber

Warm your soul with this hearty and low-sodium vegetarian minestrone soup, packed with a rainbow of veggies and wholesome whole wheat pasta.

Chicken and Vegetable Quinoa Stew

Cooking Time: 3 hours on low

Servings: 8

Ingredients:

- ❖ 1 lb boneless, skinless chicken breasts, diced.
- ❖ 1 cup quinoa, rinsed.
- ❖ 4 cups low-sodium chicken broth
- ❖ 2 carrots, sliced.
- ❖ 2 celery stalks, diced.
- ❖ 1 onion, chopped.
- ❖ 2 cloves garlic, minced.
- ❖ 1 teaspoon thyme

Instructions:

1. Place chicken, quinoa, chicken broth, carrots, celery, onion, garlic, and thyme in the slow cooker.
2. Cook on low for 3 hours.
3. Adjust seasoning if needed before serving.

Nutritional Information:

220 calories, 25g carbs, 20g protein, 4g fat, 4g fiber

Savor the comforting goodness of this chicken and vegetable quinoa stew, a protein-rich and low-sodium delight for any day.

Tomato Basil Lentil Soup

Cooking Time: 4 hours on low

Servings: 6

Ingredients:

- ❖ 1 cup dried green or brown lentils, rinsed.
- ❖ 1 can (28 oz) crushed tomatoes.
- ❖ 4 cups vegetable broth (low sodium)
- ❖ 1 onion, diced.
- ❖ 2 carrots, chopped.
- ❖ 3 cloves garlic, minced.
- ❖ 1 teaspoon dried basil

Instructions:

1. Combine lentils, crushed tomatoes, vegetable broth, onion, carrots, garlic, and basil in the slow cooker.
2. Cook on low for 4 hours.
3. Blend with an immersion blender for a smoother texture if desired.

Nutritional Information:

160 calories, 30g carbs, 10g protein, 1g fat, 8g fiber

Indulge in the classic combination of tomatoes and basil in this hearty and low-sodium lentil soup, perfect for a cozy evening.

Beef and Barley Vegetable Stew

Cooking Time: 5 hours on low

Servings: 6

Ingredients:

- ❖ 1 lb. lean beef stew meat, cubed.
- ❖ 1 cup pearl barley
- ❖ 4 cups low-sodium beef broth
- ❖ 2 potatoes, diced.
- ❖ 2 carrots, sliced.
- ❖ 1 onion, chopped.
- ❖ 2 cloves garlic, minced.
- ❖ 1 teaspoon thyme

Instructions:

1. Combine beef, barley, beef broth, potatoes, carrots, onion, garlic, and thyme in the slow cooker.
2. Cook on low for 5 hours.
3. Season with salt and pepper to taste before serving.

Nutritional Information:

280 calories, 40g carbs, 25g protein, 3g fat, 8g fiber

Experience the heartiness of beef and barley in this wholesome and low-sodium vegetable stew, a satisfying meal for chilly days.

Spicy Black-Eyed Pea Soup

Cooking Time: 4 hours on low

Servings: 8

Ingredients:

- ❖ 2 cups dried black-eyed peas, soaked overnight and drained.
- ❖ 1 lb smoked turkey sausage, sliced.
- ❖ 1 onion, diced.
- ❖ 2 bell peppers, chopped.
- ❖ 3 cloves garlic, minced.
- ❖ 1 can (14 oz) diced tomatoes, undrained.
- ❖ 1 teaspoon cayenne pepper

Instructions:

1. Combine black-eyed peas, smoked turkey sausage, onion, bell peppers, garlic, diced tomatoes, and cayenne pepper in the slow cooker.
2. Cook on low for 4 hours.
3. Adjust seasoning if needed before serving.

Nutritional Information:

240 calories, 30g carbs, 18g protein, 5g fat, 8g fiber

Add a kick to your meal with this flavorful and protein-packed spicy black-eyed pea soup, a Southern-inspired favorite.

Sweet Potato and Chickpea Curry Stew

Cooking Time: 4 hours on low

Servings: 6

Ingredients:

- ❖ 2 sweet potatoes peeled and diced.
- ❖ 2 cans (15 oz each) chickpeas drained and rinsed.
- ❖ 1 onion, chopped.
- ❖ 3 cloves garlic, minced.
- ❖ 1 can (14 oz) coconut milk (light)
- ❖ 2 tablespoons curry powder

Instructions:

1. Combine sweet potatoes, chickpeas, onion, garlic, coconut milk, and curry powder in the slow cooker.
2. Cook on low for 4 hours.
3. Serve over rice or quinoa.

Nutritional Information:

280 calories, 45g carbs, 10g protein, 8g fat, 10g fiber

Enjoy a taste of comfort with this sweet potato and chickpea curry stew, a vibrant and nutritious option for a satisfying meal.

Mushroom and Wild Rice Soup

Cooking Time: 3 hours on low

Servings: 8

Ingredients:

- ❖ 1 cup wild rice, rinsed.
- ❖ 8 cups vegetable broth (low sodium)
- ❖ 1 lb mushrooms, sliced.
- ❖ 2 carrots, diced.
- ❖ 2 celery stalks, chopped.
- ❖ 1 onion, chopped.
- ❖ 3 cloves garlic, minced.

Instructions:

1. Combine wild rice, vegetable broth, mushrooms, carrots, celery, onion, and garlic in the slow cooker.
2. Cook on low for 3 hours.
3. Season with salt and pepper to taste before serving.

Nutritional Information:

220 calories, 40g carbs, 8g protein, 3g fat, 6g fiber

Delight in the earthy flavors of mushrooms and the heartiness of wild rice in this comforting and low-sodium soup.

Turkey and Vegetable Chili

Cooking Time: 4 hours on low

Servings: 8

Ingredients:

- ❖ 1 lb ground turkey (93% lean)
- ❖ 1 onion, diced.
- ❖ 1 bell pepper, chopped.
- ❖ 2 cans (15 oz each) kidney beans drained and rinsed.
- ❖ 1 can (28 oz) crushed tomatoes.
- ❖ 2 tablespoons chili powder
- ❖ 1 teaspoon cumin

Instructions:

1. Cook ground turkey, onion, and bell pepper in a skillet until browned; transfer to the slow cooker.
2. Add kidney beans, crushed tomatoes, chili powder, and cumin.
3. Cook on low for 4 hours.

Nutritional Information:

240 calories, 30g carbs, 20g protein, 5g fat, 8g fiber

Warm up with a bowl of turkey and vegetable chili, a protein-rich and low-sodium twist on a classic comfort food.

Lemon Chicken Orzo Soup

Cooking Time: 3 hours on low

Servings: 6

Ingredients:

- ❖ 1 lb boneless, skinless chicken thighs
- ❖ 1 cup orzo pasta
- ❖ 8 cups low-sodium chicken broth
- ❖ 2 carrots, sliced.
- ❖ 2 celery stalks, diced.
- ❖ 1 onion, chopped.
- ❖ Juice of 2 lemons

Instructions:

1. Place chicken, orzo pasta, chicken broth, carrots, celery, onion, and lemon juice in the slow cooker.
2. Cook on low for 3 hours.
3. Shred chicken before serving.

Nutritional Information:

220 calories, 25g carbs, 20g protein, 4g fat, 3g fiber

Savor the brightness of lemon in this comforting and low-sodium chicken orzo soup, a soothing option for any day.

Black Bean and Vegetable Chili

Cooking Time: 4 hours on low

Servings: 8

Ingredients:

- ❖ 2 cans (15 oz each) black beans drained and rinsed.
- ❖ 1 onion, chopped.
- ❖ 2 bell peppers, diced.
- ❖ 1 zucchini, diced.
- ❖ 1 can (28 oz) crushed tomatoes.
- ❖ 2 tablespoons chili powder
- ❖ 1 teaspoon cumin

Instructions:

1. Combine black beans, onion, bell peppers, zucchini, crushed tomatoes, chili powder, and cumin in the slow cooker.
2. Cook on low for 4 hours.
3. Season with salt and pepper to taste before serving.

Nutritional Information:

180 calories, 35g carbs, 8g protein, 1g fat, 10g fiber

Delight in the richness of black beans and an array of colorful veggies in this hearty and low-sodium chili.

CHAPTER 5

POULTRY PERFECTION

Lemon Garlic Herb Chicken

Cooking Time: 4 hours on low

Servings: 4

Ingredients:

- ❖ 4 boneless, skinless chicken breasts
- ❖ 1/4 cup lemon juice
- ❖ 2 tablespoons olive oil
- ❖ 3 cloves garlic, minced.
- ❖ 1 teaspoon dried thyme
- ❖ Salt and pepper to taste

Instructions:

1. Place chicken breasts in the slow cooker.
2. In a bowl, mix lemon juice, olive oil, garlic, thyme, salt, and pepper.
3. Pour the mixture over the chicken and cook on low for 4 hours.

Nutritional Information:

250 calories, 2g carbs, 30g protein, 13g fat, 0g fiber

Infuse your poultry with the bright flavors of lemon, garlic, and herbs in this succulent and low-sodium chicken dish.

Honey Mustard Turkey Breast

Cooking Time: 5 hours on low

Servings: 6

Ingredients:

- ❖ 2 lbs turkey breast, boneless and skinless
- ❖ 1/4 cup Dijon mustard
- ❖ 2 tablespoons honey
- ❖ 1 tablespoon olive oil
- ❖ 1 teaspoon dried rosemary
- ❖ Salt and pepper to taste

Instructions:

1. Place turkey breast in the slow cooker.
2. In a bowl, mix Dijon mustard, honey, olive oil, rosemary, salt, and pepper.
3. Rub the mixture over the turkey and cook on low for 5 hours.

Nutritional Information:

180 calories, 5g carbs, 25g protein, 7g fat, 0g fiber

Elevate your turkey game with the sweet and savory combination of honey and Dijon mustard in this delightful and low-sodium recipe.

Cranberry Orange Chicken

Cooking Time: 4 hours on low

Servings: 4

Ingredients:

- ❖ 4 boneless, skinless chicken thighs
- ❖ 1 cup fresh cranberries
- ❖ 1/2 cup orange juice
- ❖ 2 tablespoons maple syrup
- ❖ 1 teaspoon cinnamon
- ❖ Salt and pepper to taste

Instructions:

1. Place chicken thighs in the slow cooker.
2. In a bowl, mix cranberries, orange juice, maple syrup, cinnamon, salt, and pepper.
3. Pour the mixture over the chicken and cook on low for 4 hours.

Nutritional Information:

220 calories, 15g carbs, 20g protein, 8g fat, 3g fiber

Celebrate the flavors of the season with this cranberry and orange-infused chicken, a festive and low-sodium dish.

Garlic Herb Turkey Meatballs

Cooking Time: 3 hours on low

Servings: 6

Ingredients:

- ❖ 1 lb ground turkey (93% lean)
- ❖ 1/2 cup breadcrumbs
- ❖ 2 cloves garlic, minced.
- ❖ 1/4 cup fresh parsley, chopped.
- ❖ 1 teaspoon dried oregano
- ❖ 1 egg

Instructions:

1. In a bowl, combine ground turkey, breadcrumbs, garlic, parsley, oregano, and egg.
2. Shape into meatballs and place in the slow cooker.
3. Cook on low for 3 hours.

Nutritional Information:

160 calories, 10g carbs, 18g protein, 6g fat, 1g fiber

Enjoy a lean and flavorful option with these garlic herb turkey meatballs, a protein-packed and low-sodium delight.

Apricot Glazed Chicken

Cooking Time: 4 hours on low

Servings: 4

Ingredients:

- ❖ 4 bone-in, skinless chicken thighs
- ❖ 1/2 cup apricot preserves (unsweetened)
- ❖ 2 tablespoons soy sauce (low sodium)
- ❖ 1 tablespoon Dijon mustard
- ❖ 1 teaspoon ginger, minced.
- ❖ Salt and pepper to taste

Instructions:

1. Place chicken thighs in the slow cooker.
2. In a bowl, mix apricot preserves, soy sauce, Dijon mustard, ginger, salt, and pepper.
3. Brush the mixture over the chicken and cook on low for 4 hours.

Nutritional Information:

240 calories, 15g carbs, 20g protein, 10g fat, 0g fiber

Experience a burst of sweetness with this apricot-glazed chicken, a delightful and low-sodium twist on classic poultry.

Lime Cilantro Chicken Tacos

Cooking Time: 3 hours on low

Servings: 6

Ingredients:

- ❖ 2 lbs. boneless, skinless chicken breasts
- ❖ Juice of 3 limes
- ❖ 1/4 cup fresh cilantro, chopped.
- ❖ 2 teaspoons ground cumin
- ❖ 1 teaspoon chili powder
- ❖ Salt and pepper to taste

Instructions:

1. Place chicken breasts in the slow cooker.
2. In a bowl, mix lime juice, cilantro, cumin, chili powder, salt, and pepper.
3. Pour the mixture over the chicken and cook on low for 3 hours.

Nutritional Information:

180 calories, 2g carbs, 25g protein, 7g fat, 0g fiber

Create a fiesta in your kitchen with these lime cilantro chicken tacos, a zesty and low-sodium option for your taco night.

Mango Coconut Curry Chicken

Cooking Time: 4 hours on low

Servings: 4

Ingredients:

- ❖ 4 boneless, skinless chicken thighs
- ❖ 1 cup mango, diced.
- ❖ 1 can (14 oz) coconut milk (light)
- ❖ 2 tablespoons curry powder
- ❖ 1 tablespoon soy sauce (low sodium)
- ❖ 1 tablespoon honey

Instructions:

1. Place chicken thighs in the slow cooker.
2. In a blender, combine mango, coconut milk, curry powder, soy sauce, and honey.
3. Pour the mixture over the chicken and cook on low for 4 hours.

Nutritional Information:

280 calories, 20g carbs, 25g protein, 12g fat, 2g fiber

Transport your taste buds to the tropics with this mango coconut curry chicken, a luscious and low-sodium slow cooker delight.

Rosemary Balsamic Chicken

Cooking Time: 4 hours on low

Servings: 4

Ingredients:

- ❖ 4 bone-in, skinless chicken breasts
- ❖ 1/4 cup balsamic vinegar
- ❖ 2 tablespoons olive oil
- ❖ 2 tablespoons fresh rosemary, chopped.
- ❖ 2 cloves garlic, minced.
- ❖ Salt and pepper to taste

Instructions:

1. Place chicken breasts in the slow cooker.
2. In a bowl, mix balsamic vinegar, olive oil, rosemary, garlic, salt, and pepper.
3. Brush the mixture over the chicken and cook on low for 4 hours.

Nutritional Information:

230 calories, 2g carbs, 25g protein, 13g fat, 0g fiber

Elevate your poultry game with the rich flavors of rosemary and balsamic vinegar in this savory and low-sodium chicken dish.

Teriyaki Pineapple Chicken

Cooking Time: 3 hours on low

Servings: 6

Ingredients:

- ❖ 2 lbs. boneless, skinless chicken thighs
- ❖ 1 cup pineapple chunks
- ❖ 1/2 cup low-sodium soy sauce
- ❖ 1/4 cup honey
- ❖ 2 teaspoons ginger, minced.
- ❖ 2 cloves garlic, minced.

Instructions:

1. Place chicken thighs in the slow cooker.
2. In a bowl, mix pineapple chunks, soy sauce, honey, ginger, and garlic.
3. Pour the mixture over the chicken and cook on low for 3 hours.

Nutritional Information:

250 calories, 20g carbs, 25g protein, 8g fat, 1g fiber

Take your taste buds on a tropical journey with this teriyaki pineapple chicken, a sweet and tangy low-sodium slow cooker sensation.

Buffalo Chicken Lettuce Wraps

Cooking Time: 4 hours on low

Servings: 4

Ingredients:

- ❖ 2 lbs. boneless, skinless chicken breasts
- ❖ 1 cup buffalo sauce (low sodium)
- ❖ 1/4 cup ranch dressing (low sodium)
- ❖ 1 teaspoon garlic powder
- ❖ 1 teaspoon onion powder
- ❖ Lettuce leaves for wrapping.

Instructions:

1. Place chicken breasts in the slow cooker.
2. In a bowl, mix buffalo sauce, ranch dressing, garlic powder, and onion powder.
3. Pour the mixture over the chicken and cook on low for 4 hours.
4. Shred the chicken and serve in lettuce wraps.

Nutritional Information:

220 calories, 2g carbs, 30g protein, 10g fat, 0g fiber

Spice up your mealtime with these buffalo chicken lettuce wraps, a protein-packed and low-sodium option for a satisfying bite.

CHAPTER 6

SEAFOOD SENSATIONS

Lemon Garlic Herb Shrimp

Cooking Time: 2 hours on low

Servings: 4

Ingredients:

- ❖ 1 lb large shrimp, peeled and deveined.
- ❖ 1/4 cup olive oil
- ❖ 3 cloves garlic, minced.
- ❖ 2 tablespoons fresh parsley, chopped.
- ❖ Juice of 2 lemons
- ❖ Salt and pepper to taste

Instructions:

1. In a bowl, mix shrimp, olive oil, garlic, parsley, lemon juice, salt, and pepper.
2. Transfer to the slow cooker and cook on low for 2 hours.

Nutritional Information:

180 calories, 2g carbs, 25g protein, 9g fat, 0g fiber

Savor the freshness of shrimp infused with the vibrant flavors of lemon, garlic, and herbs in this quick and low-sodium seafood sensation.

Coconut Curry Salmon

Cooking Time: 3 hours on low

Servings: 4

Ingredients:

- ❖ 4 salmon fillets
- ❖ 1 can (14 oz) coconut milk (light)
- ❖ 2 tablespoons curry powder
- ❖ 1 tablespoon soy sauce (low sodium)
- ❖ 1 tablespoon honey

Instructions:

1. Place salmon fillets in the slow cooker.
2. In a bowl, mix coconut milk, curry powder, soy sauce, and honey.
3. Pour the mixture over the salmon and cook on low for 3 hours.

Nutritional Information:

300 calories, 10g carbs, 25g protein, 15g fat, 1g fiber

Indulge in the richness of coconut curry with this slow-cooked salmon, a delightful and low-sodium dish that's bursting with flavor.

Garlic Butter Scallops

Cooking Time: 1.5 hours on low

Servings: 4

Ingredients:

- ❖ 1 lb. scallops
- ❖ 1/2 cup unsalted butter
- ❖ 4 cloves garlic, minced.
- ❖ 2 tablespoons fresh parsley, chopped.
- ❖ Salt and pepper to taste

Instructions:

1. In a skillet, sear scallops briefly in 1 tablespoon of butter.
2. Transfer scallops to the slow cooker and add the remaining butter and minced garlic. Sprinkle with salt, pepper, and fresh parsley.
3. Cook on low for 1.5 hours in the slow cooker.

Nutritional Information:

240 calories, 3g carbs, 20g protein, 16g fat, 0g fiber

Elevate your dining experience with these succulent garlic butter scallops, perfectly seared and slow-cooked for a melt-in-your-mouth sensation.

Tomato Basil Cod

Cooking Time: 2.5 hours on low

Servings: 4

Ingredients:

- ❖ 4 cod fillets
- ❖ 1 can (14 oz) diced tomatoes, drained.
- ❖ 1/4 cup olive oil
- ❖ 1/4 cup fresh basil, chopped.
- ❖ 2 cloves garlic, minced.
- ❖ Salt and pepper to taste

Instructions:

1. Place cod fillets in the slow cooker.
2. In a bowl, mix diced tomatoes, olive oil, basil, garlic, salt, and pepper.
3. Pour the mixture over the cod and cook on low for 2.5 hours.

Nutritional Information:

220 calories, 5g carbs, 25g protein, 12g fat, 1g fiber

Experience the taste of the Mediterranean with this tomato basil cod, slow cooked to perfection for a light and flavorful seafood dish.

Citrus Herb Tilapia

Cooking Time: 2 hours on low

Servings: 4

Ingredients:

- ❖ 4 tilapia fillets
- ❖ Juice of 2 oranges
- ❖ Juice of 1 lemon
- ❖ 2 tablespoons olive oil
- ❖ 1 teaspoon dried thyme
- ❖ Salt and pepper to taste

Instructions:

1. Place tilapia fillets in the slow cooker.
2. In a bowl, mix orange juice, lemon juice, olive oil, thyme, salt, and pepper.
3. Pour the mixture over the tilapia and cook on low for 2 hours.

Nutritional Information:

180 calories, 2g carbs, 25g protein, 9g fat, 0g fiber

Brighten up your palate with this citrus herb tilapia, a zesty and low-sodium slow cooker creation that's as refreshing as it is delicious.

Sesame Ginger Haddock

Cooking Time: 3 hours on low

Servings: 4

Ingredients:

- ❖ 4 haddock fillets
- ❖ 1/4 cup low-sodium soy sauce
- ❖ 2 tablespoons sesame oil
- ❖ 1 tablespoon rice vinegar
- ❖ 1 tablespoon fresh ginger, grated.
- ❖ 1 tablespoon sesame seeds

Instructions:

1. Place haddock fillets in the slow cooker.
2. In a bowl, mix soy sauce, sesame oil, rice vinegar, ginger, and sesame seeds.
3. Pour the mixture over the haddock and cook on low for 3 hours.

Nutritional Information:

250 calories, 3g carbs, 25g protein, 15g fat, 1g fiber

Journey to the Far East with this sesame ginger haddock, a slow-cooked seafood sensation that combines bold flavors for an unforgettable dish.

Mediterranean Shrimp Pasta

Cooking Time: 2.5 hours on low

Servings: 4

Ingredients:

- ❖ 1 lb large shrimp, peeled and deveined.
- ❖ 1 can (14 oz) artichoke hearts drained and chopped.
- ❖ 1 cup cherry tomatoes, halved.
- ❖ 1/4 cup kalamata olives, sliced.
- ❖ 2 cloves garlic, minced.
- ❖ 1 teaspoon dried oregano

Instructions:

1. In the slow cooker, combine shrimp, artichoke hearts, cherry tomatoes, olives, garlic, and oregano.
2. Cook on low for 2.5 hours.
3. Serve over your favorite low-sodium pasta or rice.

Nutritional Information:

220 calories, 10g carbs, 25g protein, 8g fat, 2g fiber

Bring the flavors of the Mediterranean to your table with this shrimp pasta, a slow-cooked delight that's both satisfying and heart-healthy.

Lime Cilantro Mahi Mahi Tacos

Cooking Time: 2 hours on low

Servings: 4

Ingredients:

- ❖ 4 mahi mahi fillets
- ❖ Juice of 3 limes
- ❖ 1/4 cup fresh cilantro, chopped.
- ❖ 1 teaspoon ground cumin
- ❖ 1 teaspoon chili powder
- ❖ Salt and pepper to taste

Instructions:

1. Place mahi mahi fillets in the slow cooker.
2. In a bowl, mix lime juice, cilantro, cumin, chili powder, salt, and pepper.
3. Pour the mixture over the mahi mahi and cook on low for 2 hours.

Nutritional Information:

240 calories, 3g carbs, 25g protein, 13g fat, 1g fiber

Add a tropical twist to your taco night with these lime cilantro mahi mahi tacos, a flavorful and low-sodium option for a festive meal.

Spicy Cajun Catfish

Cooking Time: 3 hours on low

Servings: 4

Ingredients:

- ❖ 4 catfish fillets
- ❖ 2 tablespoons Cajun seasoning (low sodium)
- ❖ 1 tablespoon olive oil
- ❖ 1 bell pepper, sliced.
- ❖ 1 onion, sliced.
- ❖ 2 celery stalks, chopped.

Instructions:

1. Rub catfish fillets with Cajun seasoning.
2. In the slow cooker, heat olive oil and add catfish, bell pepper, onion, and celery.
3. Cook on low for 3 hours.

Nutritional Information:

230 calories, 5g carbs, 25g protein, 12g fat, 2g fiber

Spice up your seafood routine with this spicy Cajun catfish, slow cooked for a tender and flavorful experience that packs a punch.

Asian Glazed Tuna Steaks

Cooking Time: 2.5 hours on low

Servings: 4

Ingredients:

- ❖ 4 tuna steaks
- ❖ 1/4 cup low-sodium soy sauce
- ❖ 2 tablespoons honey
- ❖ 1 tablespoon rice vinegar
- ❖ 1 teaspoon fresh ginger, grated.
- ❖ 1 teaspoon sesame seeds

Instructions:

1. Place tuna steaks in the slow cooker.
2. In a bowl, mix soy sauce, honey, rice vinegar, ginger, and sesame seeds.
3. Pour the mixture over the tuna steaks and cook on low for 2.5 hours.

Nutritional Information:

280 calories, 8g carbs, 30g protein, 14g fat, 1g fiber

Transport your taste buds to Asia with these Asian glazed tuna steaks, slow-cooked to perfection for a savory and low-sodium seafood sensation.

CHAPTER 7

MEATLESS MARVELS

Vegetarian Chili

Cooking Time: 4 hours on low

Servings: 6

Ingredients:

- ❖ 2 cans (15 oz each) kidney beans drained and rinsed.
- ❖ 1 can (28 oz) crushed tomatoes.
- ❖ 1 cup corn kernels (frozen or fresh)
- ❖ 1 onion, diced.
- ❖ 1 bell pepper, chopped.
- ❖ 2 cloves garlic, minced.
- ❖ 2 tablespoons chili powder

Instructions:

1. Combine kidney beans, crushed tomatoes, corn, onion, bell pepper, garlic, and chili powder in the slow cooker.
2. Cook on low for 4 hours.

Nutritional Information:

220 calories, 40g carbs, 8g protein, 3g fat, 10g fiber

Warm up with a hearty bowl of vegetarian chili, loaded with beans, vegetables, and bold spices for a satisfying and low-sodium meatless marvel.

Slow Cooker Ratatouille

Cooking Time: 3 hours on low

Servings: 4

Ingredients:

- ❖ 1 eggplant, diced.
- ❖ 2 zucchinis, sliced.
- ❖ 1 bell pepper, diced.
- ❖ 1 onion, sliced.
- ❖ 2 cloves garlic, minced.
- ❖ 1 can (14 oz) diced tomatoes.
- ❖ 1 teaspoon dried thyme

Instructions:

1. Layer eggplant, zucchinis, bell pepper, onion, and garlic in the slow cooker.
2. Pour diced tomatoes over the vegetables, sprinkle with thyme, and cook on low for 3 hours.

Nutritional Information:

120 calories, 25g carbs, 3g protein, 1g fat, 8g fiber

Enjoy the flavors of the Mediterranean with this slow cooker ratatouille, a colorful and nutritious dish that's low in sodium and high in taste.

Quinoa and Vegetable Stew

Cooking Time: 4 hours on low

Servings: 6

Ingredients:

- ❖ 1 cup quinoa, rinsed.
- ❖ 3 carrots, sliced.
- ❖ 2 celery stalks, chopped.
- ❖ 1 onion, diced.
- ❖ 2 cloves garlic, minced.
- ❖ 1 can (15 oz) chickpeas drained and rinsed.
- ❖ 8 cups vegetable broth (low sodium)

Instructions:

1. Combine quinoa, carrots, celery, onion, garlic, chickpeas, and vegetable broth in the slow cooker.
2. Cook on low for 4 hours.

Nutritional Information:

180 calories, 30g carbs, 8g protein, 3g fat, 6g fiber

Fuel your body with this protein-packed quinoa and vegetable stew, a low-sodium slow cooker marvel that's both hearty and wholesome.

Spinach and Mushroom Lasagna

Cooking Time: 3.5 hours on low

Servings: 8

Ingredients:

- ❖ 9 lasagna noodles, uncooked
- ❖ 2 cups ricotta cheese (part-skim)
- ❖ 2 cups spinach, chopped.
- ❖ 1 cup mushrooms, sliced.
- ❖ 2 cans (15 oz each) tomato sauce (low sodium)
- ❖ 2 cups mozzarella cheese, shredded.

Instructions:

1. In a bowl, mix ricotta cheese, spinach, and mushrooms.
2. Layer lasagna noodles, ricotta mixture, and tomato sauce in the slow cooker.
3. Repeat layers and top with mozzarella cheese.
4. Cook on low for 3.5 hours.

Nutritional Information:

320 calories, 40g carbs, 18g protein, 10g fat, 4g fiber

Indulge in the comfort of spinach and mushroom lasagna, a slow-cooked, low-sodium delight that's perfect for a cozy family dinner.

Curried Lentil Soup

Cooking Time: 4 hours on low

Servings: 6

Ingredients:

- ❖ 1 cup dried lentils, rinsed.
- ❖ 2 carrots, diced.
- ❖ 2 celery stalks, chopped.
- ❖ 1 onion, diced.
- ❖ 3 cloves garlic, minced.
- ❖ 1 can (14 oz) diced tomatoes.
- ❖ 4 cups vegetable broth (low sodium)
- ❖ 1 tablespoon curry powder

Instructions:

1. Combine lentils, carrots, celery, onion, garlic, diced tomatoes, vegetable broth, and curry powder in the slow cooker.
2. Cook on low for 4 hours.

Nutritional Information:

220 calories, 40g carbs, 14g protein, 1g fat, 10g fiber

Warm your soul with a bowl of curried lentil soup, a flavorful and low-sodium slow cooker marvel that's packed with plant-based protein.

Butternut Squash Risotto

Cooking Time: 3.5 hours on low

Servings: 4

Ingredients:

- ❖ 1 cup Arborio rice
- ❖ 3 cups butternut squash, diced.
- ❖ 1 onion finely chopped.
- ❖ 2 cloves garlic, minced.
- ❖ 4 cups vegetable broth (low sodium)
- ❖ 1/2 cup Parmesan cheese, grated.

Instructions:

1. In the slow cooker, combine Arborio rice, butternut squash, onion, garlic, and vegetable broth.
2. Cook on low for 3.5 hours.
3. Stir in Parmesan cheese before serving.

Nutritional Information:

280 calories, 55g carbs, 8g protein, 4g fat, 6g fiber

Indulge in the creamy goodness of butternut squash risotto, a slow-cooked, low-sodium marvel that's both comforting and elegant.

Mushroom Barley Stew

Cooking Time: 4 hours on low

Servings: 6

Ingredients:

- ❖ 1 cup barley, rinsed.
- ❖ 1 lb. mushrooms, sliced.
- ❖ 2 carrots, diced.
- ❖ 2 celery stalks, chopped.
- ❖ 1 onion, diced.
- ❖ 4 cups vegetable broth (low sodium)
- ❖ 1 teaspoon thyme

Instructions:

1. Combine barley, mushrooms, carrots, celery, onion, vegetable broth, and thyme in the slow cooker.
2. Cook on low for 4 hours.

Nutritional Information:

250 calories, 50g carbs, 8g protein, 2g fat, 10g fiber

Experience the heartiness of mushroom barley stew, a slow-cooked, low-sodium masterpiece that's rich in texture and taste.

Sweet Potato and Chickpea Curry

Cooking Time: 3 hours on low

Servings: 4

Ingredients:

- ❖ 2 sweet potatoes peeled and diced.
- ❖ 1 can (15 oz) chickpeas drained and rinsed.
- ❖ 1 onion finely chopped.
- ❖ 2 cloves garlic, minced.
- ❖ 1 can (14 oz) coconut milk (light)
- ❖ 2 tablespoons curry powder

Instructions:

1. Combine sweet potatoes, chickpeas, onion, garlic, coconut milk, and curry powder in the slow cooker.
2. Cook on low for 3 hours.

Nutritional Information:

280 calories, 45g carbs, 8g protein, 8g fat, 8g fiber

Delight your taste buds with sweet potato and chickpea curry, a slow-cooked, low-sodium dish that's both wholesome and exotic.

Caprese Quinoa Casserole

Cooking Time: 3.5 hours on low

Servings: 6

Ingredients:

- ❖ 1 cup quinoa, rinsed.
- ❖ 2 cups cherry tomatoes, halved.
- ❖ 1 lb fresh mozzarella, sliced.
- ❖ 1/2 cup fresh basil, chopped.
- ❖ 2 cloves garlic, minced.
- ❖ 2 tablespoons balsamic vinegar

Instructions:

1. Combine quinoa, cherry tomatoes, mozzarella, basil, garlic, and balsamic vinegar in the slow cooker.
2. Cook on low for 3.5 hours.

Nutritional Information:

310 calories, 35g carbs, 15g protein, 15g fat, 5g fiber

Experience the classic flavors of Caprese with this quinoa casserole, a slow-cooked, low-sodium marvel that's both elegant and satisfying.

Vegetable Coconut Curry

Cooking Time: 3 hours on low

Servings: 4

Ingredients:

- ❖ 2 cups mixed vegetables (broccoli, bell peppers, peas)
- ❖ 1 can (14 oz) coconut milk (light)
- ❖ 2 tablespoons red curry paste
- ❖ 1 tablespoon soy sauce (low sodium)
- ❖ 1 tablespoon brown sugar

Instructions:

1. Combine mixed vegetables, coconut milk, red curry paste, soy sauce, and brown sugar in the slow cooker.
2. Cook on low for 3 hours.

Nutritional Information:

230 calories, 20g carbs, 5g protein, 16g fat, 4g fiber

Savor the richness of vegetable coconut curry, a slow-cooked, low-sodium delight that's both nourishing and full of exotic flavors.

CHAPTER 8

21 DAY MEAL PLAN

Day 1:

- ❖ Breakfast: Avocado Toast
- ❖ Lunch: Vegetarian Chili
- ❖ Dinner: Mushroom Barley Stew
- ❖ Snack: Minty Watermelon Cubes

Day 2:

- ❖ Breakfast: Greek Yogurt Parfait with Berries and Honey
- ❖ Lunch: Caprese Quinoa Casserole
- ❖ Dinner: Asian Glazed Tuna Steaks
- ❖ Snack: Berry Bliss Smoothie Bowl

Day 3:

- ❖ Breakfast: Oatmeal with Sliced Peaches and Almonds
- ❖ Lunch: Quinoa and Vegetable Stew
- ❖ Dinner: Sweet Potato and Chickpea Curry
- ❖ Snack: Oatmeal Cookie Bites

Day 4:

- ❖ Breakfast: Veggie Omelette with Spinach, Mushrooms, and Feta
- ❖ Lunch: Slow Cooker Ratatouille
- ❖ Dinner: Spicy Cajun Catfish
- ❖ Snack: Citrus Burst Energizing Smoothie Bowl

Day 5:

- ❖ Breakfast: Whole Grain Pancakes with Blueberry Compote
- ❖ Lunch: Vegetable Coconut Curry
- ❖ Dinner: Lime Cilantro Mahi Mahi Tacos
- ❖ Snack: Minty Watermelon Refresher

Day 6:

- ❖ Breakfast: Greek Yogurt Bowl with Mixed Berries and Chia Seeds
- ❖ Lunch: Butternut Squash Risotto
- ❖ Dinner: Lime Garlic Herb Shrimp Pasta
- ❖ Snack: Blueberry Almond Protein Bar

Day 7:

- ❖ Breakfast: Spinach and Mushroom Breakfast Burrito
- ❖ Lunch: Curried Lentil Soup
- ❖ Dinner: Mediterranean Chickpea Salad
- ❖ Snack: Peachy Keen Protein Smoothie Bowl

Day 8:

- ❖ Breakfast: Whole Wheat Toast with Smashed Avocado and Poached Egg
- ❖ Lunch: Vegetable Coconut Curry
- ❖ Dinner: Mushroom Barley Stew
- ❖ Snack: Coconut Pineapple Green Smoothie Bowl

Day 9:

- ❖ Breakfast: Lime Cilantro Mahi Mahi Tacos
- ❖ Lunch: Quinoa and Vegetable Stew
- ❖ Dinner: Sweet Potato and Chickpea Curry
- ❖ Snack: Avocado and Tomato Salsa with Whole Grain Crackers

Day 10:

- ❖ Breakfast: Caprese Omelets with Tomatoes, Mozzarella, and Basil
- ❖ Lunch: Curried Lentil Soup
- ❖ Dinner: Asian Glazed Tuna Steaks
- ❖ Snack: Berry Bliss Smoothie Bowl

Day 11:

- ❖ Breakfast: Overnight Chia Pudding with Mixed Berries
- ❖ Lunch: Slow Cooker Ratatouille
- ❖ Dinner: Spicy Cajun Catfish
- ❖ Snack: Citrus Burst Energizing Smoothie Bowl

Day 12:

- ❖ Breakfast: Whole Grain Waffles with Sliced Peaches and Greek Yogurt
- ❖ Lunch: Butternut Squash Risotto
- ❖ Dinner: Lime Garlic Herb Shrimp Pasta
- ❖ Snack: Oatmeal Cookie Bites

Day 13:

- ❖ Breakfast: Veggie Breakfast Burrito Bowl with Quinoa
- ❖ Lunch: Spinach and Mushroom Lasagna
- ❖ Dinner: Vegetable Coconut Curry
- ❖ Snack: Blueberry Almond Protein Bar

Day 14:

- ❖ Breakfast: Greek Yogurt Parfait with Mango and Granola
- ❖ Lunch: Lime Cilantro Mahi Mahi Tacos
- ❖ Dinner: Mushroom Barley Stew
- ❖ Snack: Minty Watermelon Refresher

Day 15:

- ❖ Breakfast: Peanut Butter Banana Toast
- ❖ Lunch: Caprese Quinoa Casserole
- ❖ Dinner: Asian Glazed Tuna Steaks
- ❖ Snack: Peachy Keen Protein Smoothie Bowl

Day 16:

- ❖ Breakfast: Breakfast Burrito with Black Beans, Scrambled Eggs, and Salsa
- ❖ Lunch: Curried Lentil Soup
- ❖ Dinner: Sweet Potato and Chickpea Curry
- ❖ Snack: Oatmeal Cookie Smoothie Bowl

Day 17:

- ❖ Breakfast: Whole Wheat Bagel with Cream Cheese, Smoked Salmon, and Capers
- ❖ Lunch: Quinoa and Vegetable Stew
- ❖ Dinner: Spicy Cajun Catfish
- ❖ Snack: Citrus Burst Energizing Smoothie Bowl

Day 18:

- ❖ Breakfast: Overnight Oats with Almond Butter and Banana Slices
- ❖ Lunch: Butternut Squash Risotto
- ❖ Dinner: Lime Garlic Herb Shrimp Pasta
- ❖ Snack: Avocado Kale Power Smoothie Bowl

Day 19:

- ❖ Breakfast: Greek Yogurt Bowl with Kiwi, Pineapple, and Chia Seeds
- ❖ Lunch: Slow Cooker Ratatouille
- ❖ Dinner: Vegetable Coconut Curry
- ❖ Snack: Berry Bliss Smoothie Bowl

Day 20:

- ❖ Breakfast: Breakfast Quesadilla with Spinach, Feta, and Tomatoes
- ❖ Lunch: Lime Cilantro Mahi Mahi Tacos
- ❖ Dinner: Mushroom Barley Stew
- ❖ Snack: Coconut Pineapple Green Smoothie Bowl

Day 21:

- ❖ Breakfast: Whole Grain English Muffin with Scrambled Eggs and Sautéed Spinach
- ❖ Lunch: Caprese Quinoa Casserole
- ❖ Dinner: Asian Glazed Tuna Steaks
- ❖ Snack: Oatmeal Cookie Bites

CONCLUSION

As we reach the final pages of "Savoring Life: A Journey to Wellness with Lorene's Low Sodium Slow Cooker Cookbook," my heart is brimming with gratitude and excitement. I hope this culinary odyssey has ignited a spark within you, inspiring a newfound appreciation for the profound connection between nourishing our bodies and indulging our taste buds.

In these pages, we've shared stories of triumph over health challenges, celebrated the joy of crafting flavorful dishes, and embarked on a collective journey toward a healthier, more vibrant life. Your presence in this journey has made it all the more meaningful, and for that, I thank you from the depths of my heart.

As you close the cover of this cookbook, I encourage you to carry its essence into your kitchen and, more importantly, into your life. Let the aromas, flavors, and stories linger in your heart, becoming a guiding light on your path to wellness. Each recipe is not just a set of instructions; it's an invitation to savor life fully, to embrace the beauty of balance, and to revel in the joy of mindful eating.

Your feedback is invaluable to me, dear readers. I would love to hear about your experiences, the moments of culinary delight, and the positive changes you've witnessed in your health. Your stories have the power to inspire others on their journey to wellness, creating a ripple effect of positivity and transformation.

Do you have a favorite recipe that became a staple in your home? How has this cookbook influenced your approach to cooking and eating? Share your thoughts, your challenges, and your victories. Your feedback will not only shape future editions but will also serve as a source of motivation for those just beginning their adventure with low-sodium slow cooking.

Connect with me through social media, send me an email, or even write a heartfelt review. Your words are a testament to the community we've built, bound together by a shared commitment to health, happiness, and the sheer joy of savoring life.

As we part ways for now, remember that the journey to wellness is ongoing. May your kitchen continue to be a place of creativity, healing, and joy. May each meal you prepare be a celebration of life's abundance, a symphony of flavors that nourish not only your body but also your spirit.

Thank you for entrusting me with a small part of your culinary voyage. Here's to your health, happiness, and the many delicious moments that lie ahead.

BONUS CHAPTER

SMOOTHIES

Tropical Paradise Smoothie

Preparation Time: 5 minutes

Servings: 2

Ingredients:

- ❖ 1 cup pineapple chunks (frozen)
- ❖ 1/2 cup mango chunks (frozen)
- ❖ 1 banana
- ❖ 1 cup coconut water (unsweetened)
- ❖ 1 tablespoon chia seeds

Instructions:

1. Blend pineapple, mango, banana, coconut water, and chia seeds until smooth.

Nutritional Information:

180 calories, 40g carbs, 2g protein, 2g fat, 8g fiber

Escape to a tropical paradise with this refreshing smoothie, a low-sodium blend of exotic fruits and hydrating coconut water.

Berry Bliss Smoothie

Preparation Time: 5 minutes

Servings: 2

Ingredients:

- ❖ 1 cup mixed berries (strawberries, blueberries, raspberries)
- ❖ 1/2 cup Greek yogurt (plain, low-fat)
- ❖ 1 tablespoon honey
- ❖ 1/2 cup almond milk (unsweetened)
- ❖ Ice cubes (optional)

Instructions:

2. Blend mixed berries, Greek yogurt, honey, and almond milk until smooth.
3. Add ice cubes if desired and blend again.

Nutritional Information:

150 calories, 25g carbs, 7g protein, 3g fat, 5g fiber

Indulge in the sweetness of berries with this luscious smoothie, a low sodium treat packed with antioxidants and probiotics.

Green Goddess Detox Smoothie

Preparation Time: 7 minutes

Servings: 2

Ingredients:

- ❖ 2 cups spinach (fresh)
- ❖ 1/2 cucumber peeled and sliced.
- ❖ 1 green apple cored and chopped.
- ❖ 1/2 lemon, juiced.
- ❖ 1 cup water (filtered)

Instructions:

1. Blend spinach, cucumber, green apple, lemon juice, and water until smooth.

Nutritional Information:

70 calories, 18g carbs, 2g protein, 0g fat, 4g fiber

Revitalize your body with the Green Goddess Detox Smoothie, a low-sodium elixir that nourishes and cleanses with vibrant green ingredients.

Peachy Keen Protein Smoothie

Preparation Time: 6 minutes

Servings: 2

Ingredients:

- ❖ 1 cup peaches (frozen)
- ❖ 1/2 cup cottage cheese (low-fat)
- ❖ 1/2 cup almond milk (unsweetened)
- ❖ 1 tablespoon flaxseeds
- ❖ 1 teaspoon vanilla extract

Instructions:

1. Blend peaches, cottage cheese, almond milk, flaxseeds, and vanilla extract until creamy.

Nutritional Information:

220 calories, 30g carbs, 12g protein, 6g fat, 5g fiber

Fuel your day with the Peachy Keen Protein Smoothie, a low-sodium blend that combines the sweetness of peaches with a protein punch.

Citrus Burst Energizing Smoothie

Preparation Time: 5 minutes

Servings: 2

Ingredients:

- ❖ 1 orange peeled and segmented.
- ❖ 1/2 grapefruit peeled and segmented.
- ❖ 1 banana
- ❖ 1/2 cup Greek yogurt (plain, low-fat)
- ❖ 1/2 cup water (filtered)

Instructions:

1. Blend orange, grapefruit, banana, Greek yogurt, and water until smooth.

Nutritional Information:

160 calories, 35g carbs, 7g protein, 1g fat, 5g fiber

Awaken your senses with the Citrus Burst Energizing Smoothie, a low-sodium blend that combines the zing of citrus fruits with creamy Greek yogurt.

Minty Watermelon Refresher

Preparation Time: 5 minutes

Servings: 2

Ingredients:

- ❖ 2 cups watermelon, cubed.
- ❖ 1/2 cup cucumber, sliced.
- ❖ 1 tablespoon fresh mint leaves
- ❖ 1/2 lime, juiced.
- ❖ Ice cubes

Instructions:

1. Blend watermelon, cucumber, mint leaves, and lime juice until refreshing.
2. Add ice cubes and blend again for an extra chill.

Nutritional Information:

80 calories, 20g carbs, 1g protein, 0g fat, 2g fiber

Stay cool with the Minty Watermelon Refresher, a low-sodium smoothie that hydrates and invigorates with the essence of watermelon and mint.

Oatmeal Cookie Smoothie

Preparation Time: 6 minutes

Servings: 2

Ingredients:

- ❖ 1/2 cup rolled oats.
- ❖ 1 banana
- ❖ 2 tablespoons almond butter
- ❖ 1/2 teaspoon cinnamon
- ❖ 1 cup almond milk (unsweetened)

Instructions:

1. Blend rolled oats, banana, almond butter, cinnamon, and almond milk until creamy.

Nutritional Information:

280 calories, 35g carbs, 8g protein, 12g fat, 6g fiber

Satisfy your cravings guilt-free with the Oatmeal Cookie Smoothie, a low-sodium blend that captures the flavors of a classic treat.

Avocado Kale Power Smoothie

Preparation Time: 7 minutes

Servings: 2

Ingredients:

- ❖ 1/2 avocado peeled and pitted.
- ❖ 1 cup kale leaves, stems removed.
- ❖ 1 green apple cored and chopped.
- ❖ 1/2 lemon, juiced.
- ❖ 1 cup coconut water (unsweetened)

Instructions:

1. Blend avocado, kale, green apple, lemon juice, and coconut water until smooth.

Nutritional Information:

210 calories, 30g carbs, 4g protein, 10g fat, 8g fiber

Empower your day with the Avocado Kale Power Smoothie, a low-sodium powerhouse that combines creamy avocado with nutrient-packed kale.

Blueberry Almond Protein Smoothie

Preparation Time: 5 minutes

Servings: 2

Ingredients:

- ❖ 1 cup blueberries (frozen)
- ❖ 1/2 cup Greek yogurt (plain, low-fat)
- ❖ 2 tablespoons almond butter
- ❖ 1 cup almond milk (unsweetened)
- ❖ 1 tablespoon hemp seeds

Instructions:

1. Blend blueberries, Greek yogurt, almond butter, almond milk, and hemp seeds until rich and smooth.

Nutritional Information:

250 calories, 25g carbs, 10g protein, 14g fat, 6g fiber

Fuel your body with the Blueberry Almond Protein Smoothie, a low-sodium blend that combines the sweetness of blueberries with the richness of almond butter.

Coconut Pineapple Green Smoothie

Preparation Time: 6 minutes

Servings: 2

Ingredients:

- ❖ 1 cup pineapple chunks (frozen)
- ❖ 1 cup spinach leaves
- ❖ 1/2 banana
- ❖ 1/2 cup coconut milk (unsweetened)
- ❖ 1 tablespoon chia seeds

Instructions:

1. Blend pineapple, spinach, banana, coconut milk, and chia seeds until a vibrant green smoothie is achieved.

Nutritional Information:

200 calories, 30g carbs, 4g protein, 9g fat, 8g fiber

Transport yourself to the tropics with the Coconut Pineapple Green Smoothie, a low-sodium concoction that brings together the goodness of coconut and pineapple.

MEAL PLANNER JOURNAL

WEEKLY PLANNER

MONDAY	TUESDAY

WEDNESDAY	THURSDAY

FRIDAY	SATUREDAY

SUNDAY	NOTE

WEEKLY PLANNER

MONDAY

TUESDAY

WEDNESDAY

THURSDAY

FRIDAY

SATUREDAY

SUNDAY

NOTE

WEEKLY PLANNER

MONDAY

TUESDAY

WEDNESDAY

THURSDAY

FRIDAY

SATUREDAY

SUNDAY

NOTE

WEEKLY PLANNER

MONDAY

TUESDAY

WEDNESDAY

THURSDAY

FRIDAY

SATUREDAY

SUNDAY

NOTE

WEEKLY PLANNER

MONDAY	TUESDAY

WEDNESDAY	THURSDAY

FRIDAY	SATUREDAY

SUNDAY	NOTE

WEEKLY PLANNER

MONDAY	TUESDAY

WEDNESDAY	THURSDAY

FRIDAY	SATUREDAY

SUNDAY	NOTE

WEEKLY PLANNER

MONDAY	TUESDAY

WEDNESDAY	THURSDAY

FRIDAY	SATUREDAY

SUNDAY	NOTE

WEEKLY PLANNER

MONDAY	TUESDAY

WEDNESDAY	THURSDAY

FRIDAY	SATUREDAY

SUNDAY	NOTE

WEEKLY PLANNER

MONDAY	TUESDAY

WEDNESDAY	THURSDAY

FRIDAY	SATUREDAY

SUNDAY	NOTE

WEEKLY PLANNER

MONDAY	TUESDAY

WEDNESDAY	THURSDAY

FRIDAY	SATUREDAY

SUNDAY	NOTE

www.ingramcontent.com/pod-product-compliance
Lightning Source LLC
Chambersburg PA
CBHW082219290526
45794CB00009B/3599